ICKY PICKY SUZIE

Story by Kim Korb and Erin Leigh Quereau,

Illustrated by Joshua and Owen Korb.

Suzie didn't like yogurt.

She didn't like carrots.

She wouldn't eat corn.

She didn't like celery, cucumbers,

or any other food

starting with the letter "C".

Suzie didn't even like chocolate!

All she wanted was pizza and peanut butter.

Well, at least that's what Suzie thought.

Because she never tried any other foods.

You see, Suzie was really

picky!

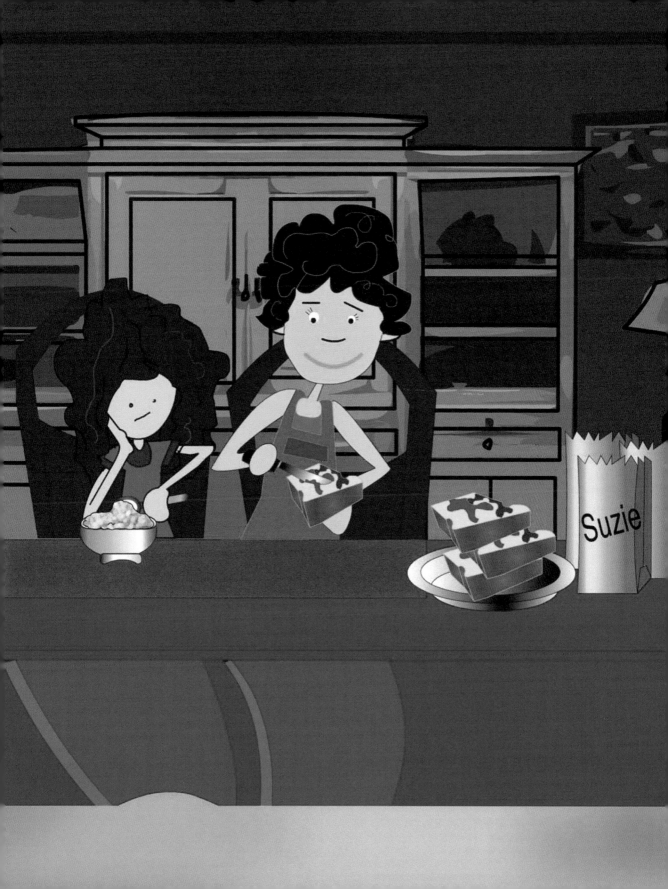

Her brothers called her a chicken
because she wouldn't try
any new foods...

Suzie stuck out her tongue and said,

"I don't even like chicken!"

Her brothers asked,
"But how do you know?
You're looking at foods with your eyes
instead of tasting them."

Suzie just walked away.

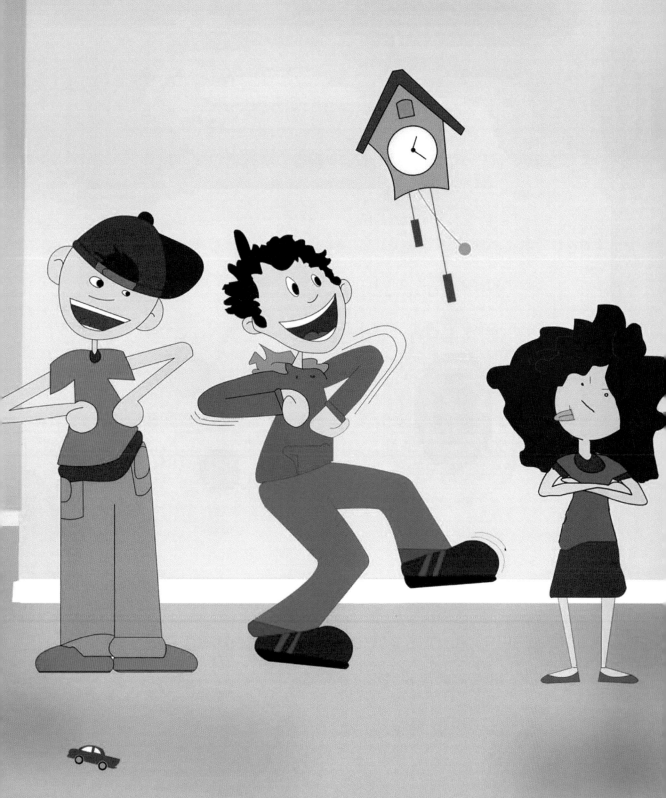

Every day in the school cafeteria,
Suzie's classmates traded snacks.
Friends tried to get Suzie to taste new foods.

They pleaded, "Hey Suzie, carrots keep your skin
soft, and make your hair shine.
Take a bite. I'll bet you'll love them."

"Hey Suzie, want a piece of my orange?
My mom says it's full of vitamin C.
It keeps you from getting sick,
and it tastes so good!"

"Suzie, want some grapes?
I bet you didn't know that they
dry them to make raisins!"

good grades

Aa Bb Cc Dd Ee Ff Gg Hh I

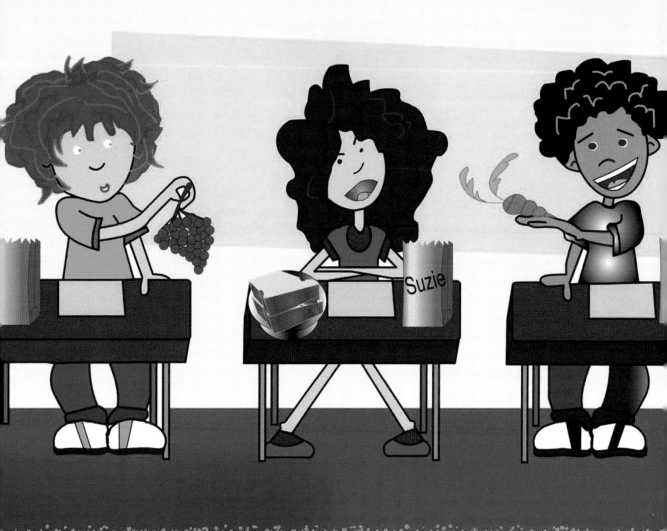

But the harder they tried,
the more Suzie would shout,

"No."

"GROSS!

GROSS!

GROSS!"

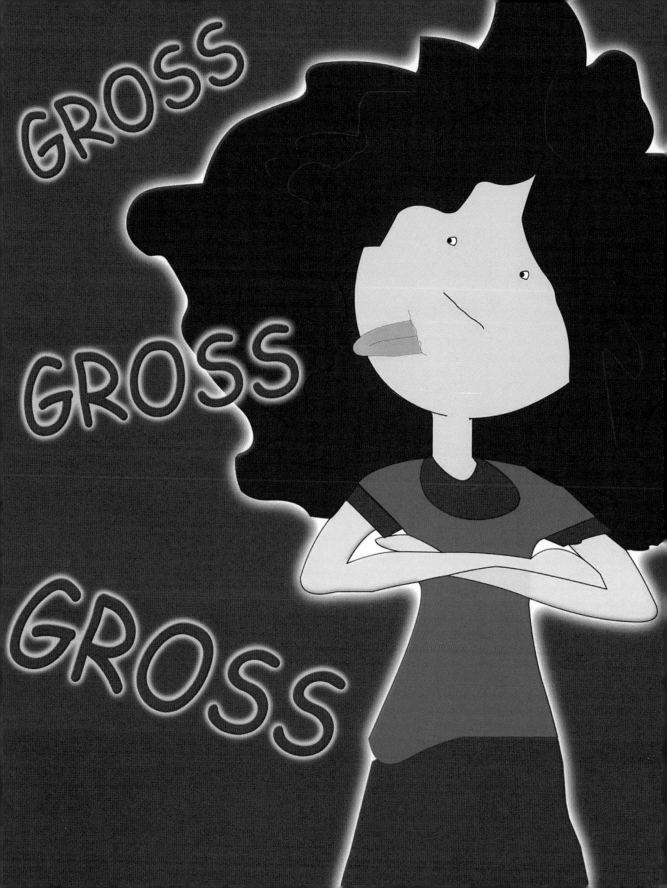

One night, Suzie had a strange dream.

In her dream, there were veggies and fruits
of all different sizes and colors.

It was so beautiful.

She didn't recognize all of the foods,
but some were the snacks her friends offered
her every day at school.

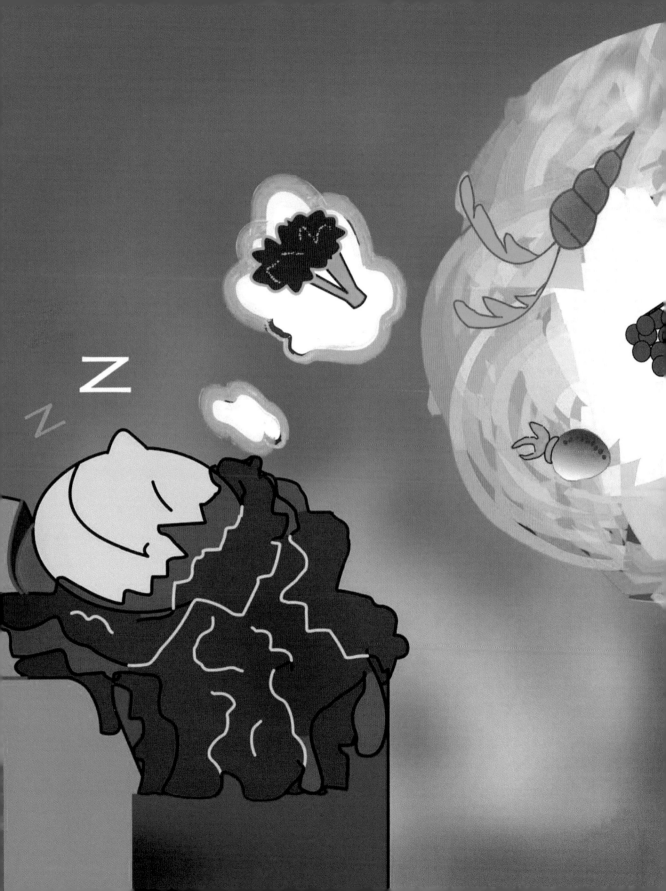

As she was dreaming,
she realized she was in a beautiful garden.

She wanted to try everything,
the fruits and vegetables looked so good.

Suzie took a bite.
"Mmmmmm!" She said.

She reached for another, and another.
Everything tasted delicious!

Suzie was trying new foods
and...and...

...and she liked them!

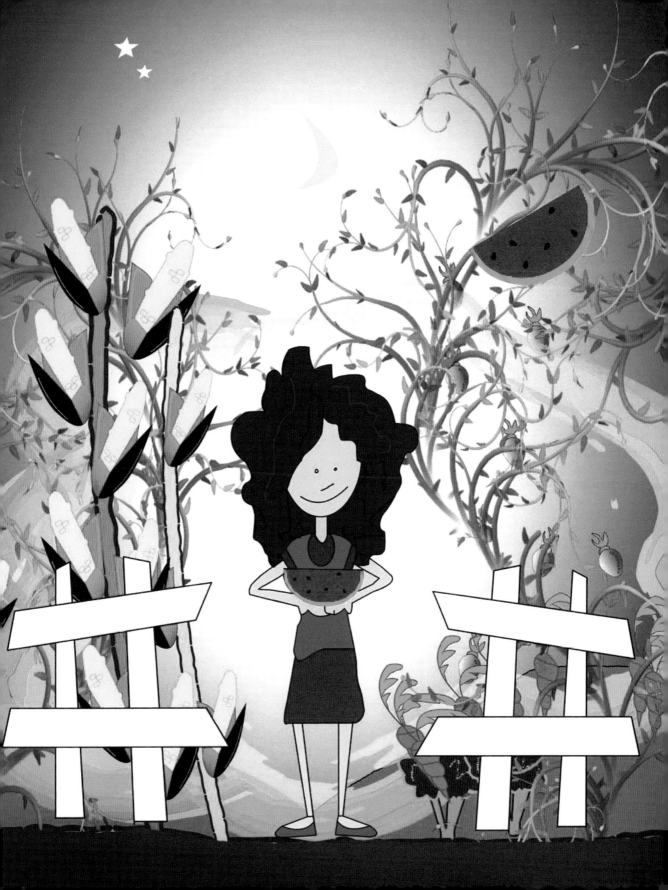

In the morning, Suzie woke up
with a huge smile on her face.

She felt different.

She felt BRAVE!!!

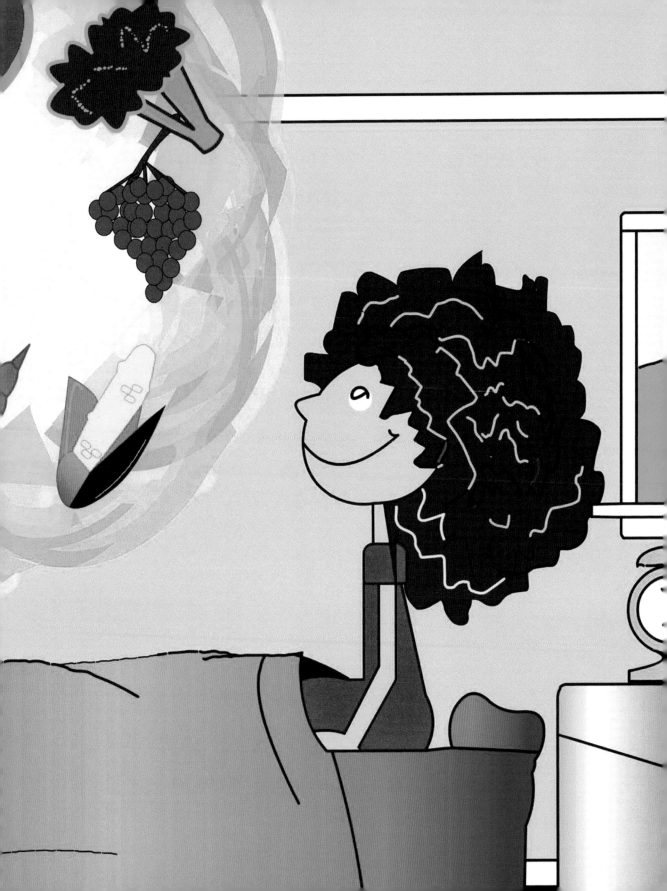

That day, at snack time, a chef
was preparing a special treat for Suzie's class...
WATERMELON!

The chef cut the green, oval fruit
into slices and placed one slice
on each student's desk.
Suzie looked down at the green and red slice.

She quickly pushed it aside, folded her arms,
and pouted "EWWWW!"

"Mmmmmmmm!" someone said.

"Come on, Suzie, try just a little bite."

"NO!" said Suzie.

"NO...NO...NO...!"

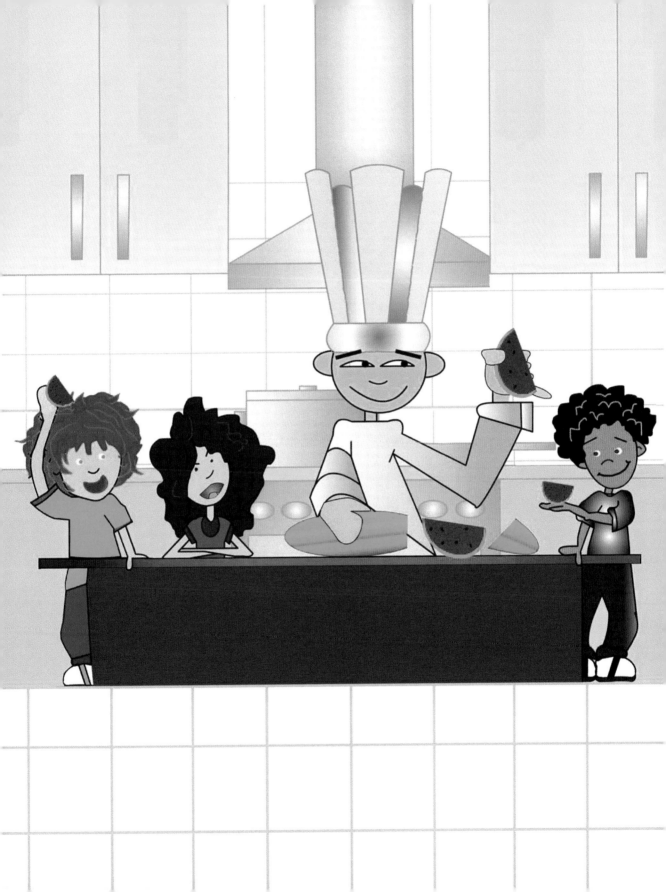

But then,
Suzie remembered her dream.

She picked up the watermelon,
closed her eyes and took a bite.

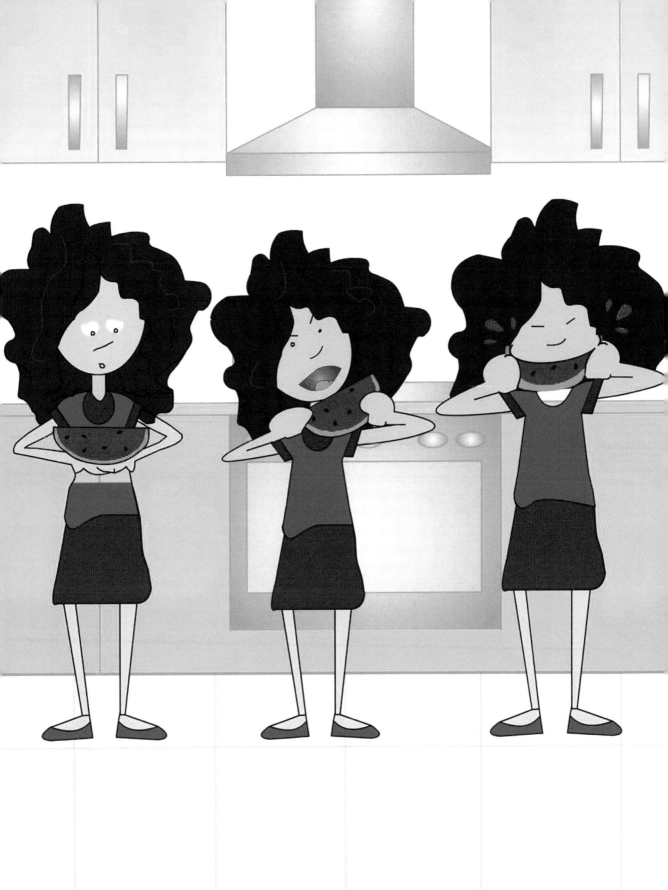

Suzie smiled and thought,
this is so sweet and juicy!

She took another bite.

Her whole class began to cheer
and clap their hands.

"HORRAY FOR SUZIE!"
they shouted.

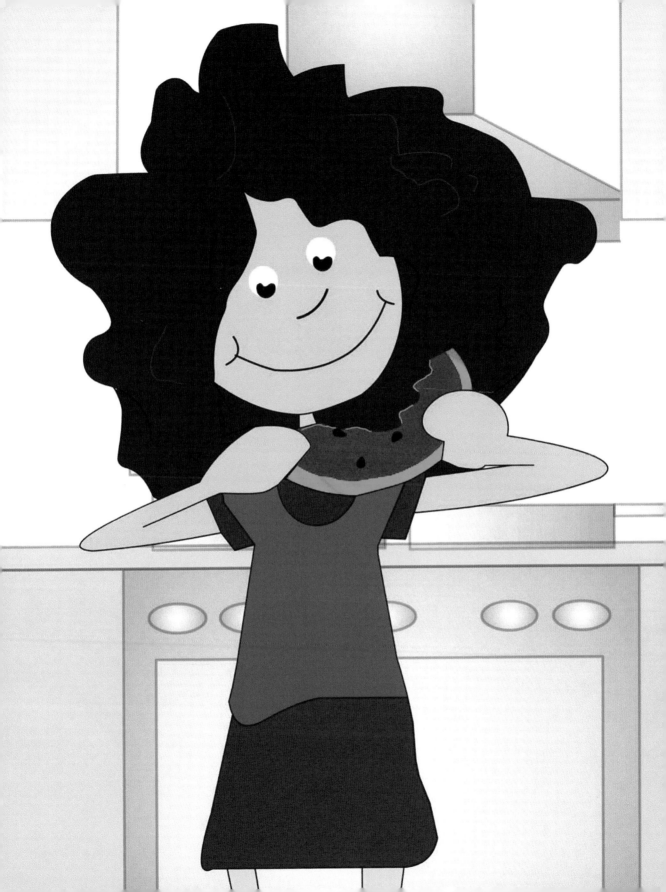

From that day on,
Suzie never turned down any new foods.

She would try new foods
every time they were offered.

Her mom and dad were proud of her
and her brothers never again
called her "chicken."

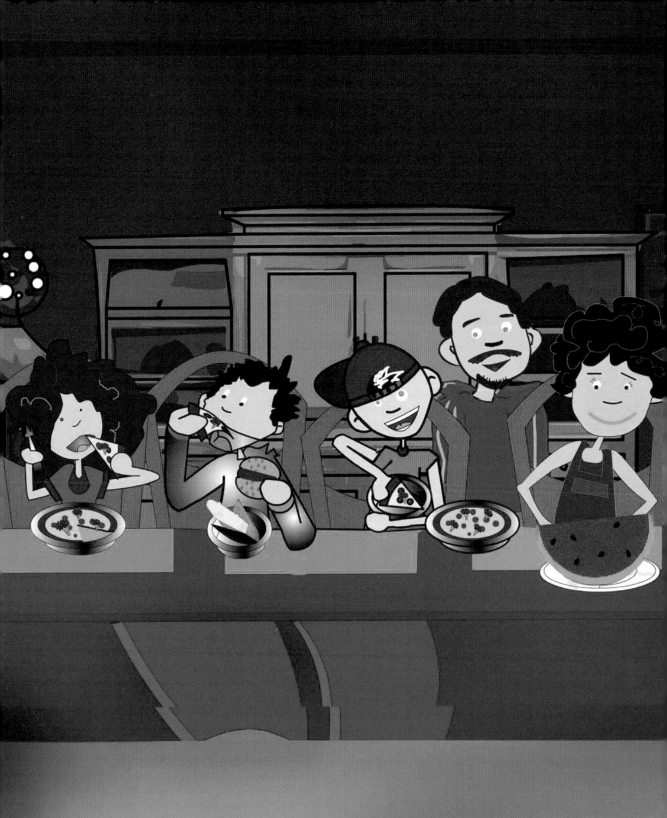

Now, Suzie was the one asking her new friends
to try her snacks at lunch time.

And, when one of them folded their arms
and pouted saying "GROSS!",
Suzie just looked at them, smiled and said,
"You will love it.

Oh, come on
and don't be so
Icky Picky!"

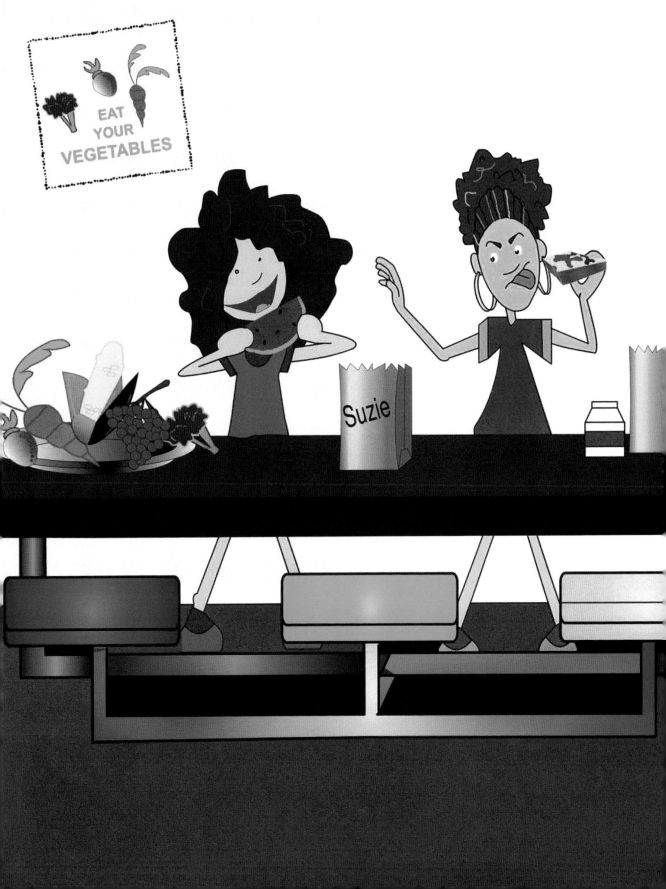

Acknowledgments

I want to thank my loving (and creative) family, for without their help this story would have stayed inside my head.

It was a family project for 10 years, a collaboration (a Korboration, if you will) until my daughter, Erin, helped get the words of my story onto paper.

My sons, Owen and Josh, used their incredible talents to bring Suzie to life with illustrations that made Suzie come alive.

My husband Ed, our backbone, helped with all our tasks and kept us going to make this book a reality.

Thanks also to the Rhode Island students and teachers, who loved the story, asked for it, and encouraged me to publish this story.

Kids First/Farm Fresh RI, non-profit agencies, that gave me the platform to tell this story and encourage children to try new foods.

My neighbor and friend Michael Grossman of the ebookbakery.com, gave me that much needed push to send Suzie out into the world.

I couldn't have done this without each of you, and for that I am truly grateful!

About the Author

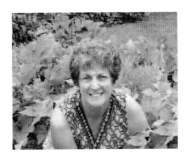

 Kim Korb's classes on gardening, cooking and nutrition have for years encouraged picky New England grade school children to understand where good food comes from and to try fresh veggies and fruit.

Kim discovered early on that a surprising number of kids know only that food comes from supermarkets. In her workshops, Kim shows the children seeds,plants,flowers,stems,leaves,fruits and roots. Let Kim tell you in her own words:

"We began with a gardening program to show how a seed, when planted, grows into a large plant, and the plant is not only edible, it's delicious and healthy for you.

I would cut up and serve them raw vegetables with a spoonful of dip: peas, lettuce, carrots, broccoli, spinach, and celery.

But there would always be some kids who thought raw foods were gross and would not try them. They were missing out on the best that nature offers, and I wanted to encourage them to try fresh vegetables. *Icky Picky Suzie* is the story that came out of my experiences.

The students could relate to Suzie. They wrote me letters thanking me for sharing that story and how it helped them to try new fruits and veggies.

"These days the Korb family, like most, is spread across the USA. But we often get together with our kids at the family home in Rhode Island and eat fresh food from our garden, just as our kids did when they were growing up (Well, after they got over being icky picky!).

"*Icky Picky Suzie* is a family collaboration that is 10 years in the making! We really enjoyed making this book a reality!"

22898429R00018

Made in the USA
Charleston, SC
03 October 2013